Lose Live

By: Ron Irwin

Copyright © 2015 Ron Irwin

Cover Photo by:

Harvey Branman

i

Other Books by
Ron Irwin

The FAA Will Kill You

Geezer and the Kid: Adventures in Flight

Manfred Moose Flies to Hong Kong

One and a Half Pinoy

Live Die Live Again

California Coast

Procrastinator's Bible

Hollywood on Stage: A critical review

Hell's Bank

Table of Contents

It Ain't About Fashion

Before I delve into the reasons why we all must combat obesity and offer proven ways to win the battle I want to make it abundantly clear that losing weight is by far most important for very real and very serious health reasons and NOT for fashion. It seems like darn near everyone at some point gets caught up in the desire to shed some pounds primarily for vanity reasons. In many if not most cases the perceived need is relatively small say somewhere between 10 and 30 pounds and is driven largely by a touch of vanity. The women may want to get into that size 2 dress for their next major social event so that they shine at the ball so to speak. Guys tend to be less concerned about weight issues and are often even accepting of beer bellies and other signs of poor diet but they may well want to exchange muscle for fat so that they look more buff, yet another ego driven force. This will led them to the many fad diets that can and do offer some limited short term benefit.

Fashion or ego is how the fad diets thrive. Sure enough follow pretty much any fad diet and you will most likely lose a little weight. But the moment you get at or near your desired goal the diet stops and you rapidly regain the weight plus 20%. You have now started the yoyo effect and that is a very tough situation both physically and mentally. "What is the point" you may wonder in exasperation. I follow the diet which is very tough and painful, I lose the weight or at least most of the weight and then it just comes right back with a bonus. Damn!

The same thing applies to all of the various supplements that are marketed for weight reduction, Read the labels on those supplement bottles and what you will find for the most part is a list of vitamins and maybe a few potentially helpful components such as fiber. But look at the claims. "This product when taken together with a proper diet and exercise may help reduce weight" is a stereotypical claim on virtually everyone of these so called weight loss pills. Well hell a proper diet and some exercise will indeed result in weight loss without the pill so what is the point? The only thing these pills are sure to reduce is your bank account. Now having said that I will acknowledge one small value that they do offer.

That is that while taking these weight loss supplements you are actually paying attention to your diet and exercise. Doing that will make you a wee bit more aware at least of the major transgressions such that you will be less likely to eat the whole pizza and wash it down with a few beers. Taking the pills will bring you a tiny bit more into focus but it falls far short of a real and long term solution.

So sure we all want to look and feel better and sometimes that requires a bit of weight loss. But if you are sick and tired of the yoyo effect and you are finally ready to make permanent and positive modifications in your total lifestyle read on. Taking charge and making long term positive changes becomes much easier once you fully understand the true depth of what is involved. Getting trimmed down for the prom is understandable but making critical life changes that can and will bring you to a longer, stronger and healthier life is vastly more important. To accomplish this you must first fully understand and accept the problem. That is to say you must completely and openly own your weight problem and you must also become totally aware of just how important taking charge is. To do that you need to know just how dangerous obesity can be to your life. It is far more than merely needing to switch to a larger dress size or switch over to the "big men's" section for your next clothing purchase. The truth is uncontrolled obesity can indeed kill you. So this is not about fashion, it is solidly about life. So next I will address briefly the need to own the issue and then explain in reasonable detail how doing so can not only make you stronger and healthier but may very literally save your life.

First Own the Problem

Most people spend most of their time and energy finding cleaver ways to ignore all manner of serious problems. It is a well-established but frequently deadly habit of self-deception. For purposes of this book I will focus solely on the matter of obesity because it is a massive problem that is sweeping the world and its consequences are often devastating and even deadly. Even worse as the problem mushrooms so grows the barriers of self-deception for in our modern times the notion of political correctness has engulfed our world.

In the "good old days" if you were clearly obese your friends would aggressively let you know. "Hey lard ass, how ya doin'" "Holy crap dude, where do you get your clothes, from Omar the tent maker?" There were, and still are a broad range of ways to slam at someone's condition of obesity but not these days. In our modern enlightened times we must be sensitive and not offend other people. Never be judgmental or in any way hurtful. So rather than perhaps jarring someone into recognizing and actually dealing with a potentially deadly condition we aid and abate them in their deep denial making it all that much easier for our friends and love ones to remain on path of self-destruction.

Well if the concept of political correctness has muzzled our friends then it is absolutely essential that we all take charge and be honest with ourselves. Yes the process at first will be very uncomfortable but as you set off on this path always keep in mind that what you are doing is merely taking ownership of the problem so that you can and will make it go away for real.

Let's start with a reasonably cogent definition of obesity. It can be a somewhat vague and imprecise science but there are measures and they must be at the very least looked at seriously. One approach is to define obesity by using body mass index. Here is how the Mayo Clinic states the matter:

Obesity is diagnosed when your body mass index (BMI) is 30 or higher. Your body mass index is calculated by dividing your weight in kilograms (kg) by your height in meters (m) squared.

BMI	Weight status
Below 18.5	Underweight
18.5-24.9	Normal
25.0-29.9	Overweight
30.0-34.9	Obese (Class I)
35.0-39.9	Obese (Class II)
40.0 and higher	Extreme obesity (Class III)

For most people, BMI provides a reasonable estimate of body fat. However, BMI doesn't directly measure body fat, so some people, such as muscular athletes, may have a BMI in the obese category even though they don't have excess body fat. Ask your doctor if your BMI is a problem.

Of course there is also the matter of just exactly how do you measure Body Mass Index [BMI]. Most people don't have a clue nor is it an essential measurement. But if BMI does move you then by all means get on over to your physician and have your BMI scientifically determined, Or you can look at a different measure generally known as "ideal weight." That is a chart or graph that determines the parameters of weight based upon your height and gender. Here is one such chart.

One of many height weight charts may be found at: http://www.healthchecksystems.com/heightweightchart. htm.

This one is from Health Check Systems and it is a reasonable guide. It is of necessity replete with vagaries such as exactly what is your "frame size." Yes, it offers guidance on correctly determining you frame size but there is still wiggle room and that's okay. Just use this chart as intended and it will be very useful.

Let's say for example that you are a female 5 feet 2 inches tall. The range from small to large frame type is 108 to 143 pounds. If you fall within that range you are most likely in decent shape basic health wise even though that is 35 pound range. You may still want to shed a few pounds if you are close to the 143 pound marker and especially if you believe that you are of a smaller frame size. Doing so will improve your overall health and your appearance and could very well add a wee bit of extra energy. But this is in the area of a fine adjustment and while still important not nearly as much so as when you are well beyond the high end of the range.

For example let's say you are a female 5 feet 2 inches tall and you weigh in at 165 pounds. Now that is undeniable obesity and that becomes a serious health risk. Just keep in mind that there really is no such thing as a truly perfect score as there really is no such thing as a truly perfect human being. But when you are clearly well out of the acceptable range what you are doing is putting yourself at ever increasing risk of health problems that you do not want. Allow me to acquaint you with a few of those health problems that obesity can bring to you.

Coronary Heart Disease

As your body mass index rises, so does your risk for coronary heart disease (CHD). CHD is a condition in which a waxy substance called plaque (plak) builds up inside the coronary arteries. These arteries supply oxygen-rich blood to your heart.

Plaque can narrow or block the coronary arteries and reduce blood flow to the heart muscle. This can cause angina or a heart attack. (Angina is chest pain or discomfort.)

Obesity also can lead to heart failure. This is a serious condition in which your heart can't pump enough blood to meet your body's needs.

High Blood Pressure

Blood pressure is the force of blood pushing against the walls of the arteries as the heart pumps blood. If this pressure rises and stays high over time, it can damage the body in many ways.

Your chances of having high blood pressure are greater if you're overweight or obese.

Stroke

Being overweight or obese can lead to a buildup of plaque in your arteries. Eventually, an area of plaque can rupture, causing a blood clot to form.

If the clot is close to your brain, it can block the flow of blood and oxygen to your brain and cause a stroke. The risk of having a stroke rises as BMI increases.

Type 2 Diabetes

Diabetes is a disease in which the body's blood glucose, or blood sugar, level is too high. Normally, the body breaks down food into glucose and then carries it to cells throughout the body. The cells use a hormone called insulin to turn the glucose into energy.

In type 2 diabetes, the body's cells don't use insulin properly. At first, the body reacts by making more insulin. Over time, however, the body can't make enough insulin to control its blood sugar level.

Diabetes is a leading cause of early death, CHD, stroke, kidney disease, and blindness. Most people who have type 2 diabetes are overweight.

Abnormal Blood Fats

If you're overweight or obese, you're at increased risk of having abnormal levels of blood fats. These include high levels of triglycerides and LDL ("bad") cholesterol and low levels of HDL ("good") cholesterol.

Abnormal levels of these blood fats are a risk factor for CHD. For more information about triglycerides and LDL and HDL cholesterol, go to the Health Topics High Blood Cholesterol article.

Metabolic Syndrome

Metabolic syndrome is the name for a group of risk factors that raises your risk for heart disease and other health problems, such as diabetes and stroke.

You can develop any one of these risk factors by itself, but they tend to occur together. A diagnosis of metabolic syndrome is made if you have at least three of the following risk factors:

- A large waistline. This is called abdominal obesity or "having an apple shape." Having extra fat in the waist area is a greater risk factor for CHD than having extra fat in other parts of the body, such as on the hips.
- A higher than normal triglyceride level (or you're on medicine to treat high triglycerides).
- A lower than normal HDL cholesterol level (or you're on medicine to treat low HDL cholesterol).
- Higher than normal blood pressure (or you're on medicine to treat high blood pressure).
- Higher than normal fasting blood sugar (or you're on medicine to treat diabetes).

Cancer

Being overweight or obese raises your risk for colon, breast, endometrial, and gallbladder cancers.

Osteoarthritis

Osteoarthritis is a common joint problem of the knees, hips, and lower back. The condition occurs if the tissue that protects the joints wears away. Extra weight can put more pressure and wear on joints, causing pain.

Sleep Apnea

Sleep apnea is a common disorder in which you have one or more pauses in breathing or shallow breaths while you sleep.

A person who has sleep apnea may have more fat stored around the neck. This can narrow the airway, making it hard to breathe.

Obesity Hypoventilation Syndrome

Obesity hypoventilation syndrome (OHS) is a breathing disorder that affects some obese people. In OHS, poor breathing results in too much carbon dioxide (hypoventilation) and too little oxygen in the blood (hypoxemia).

OHS can lead to serious health problems and may even cause death.

Reproductive Problems

Obesity can cause menstrual issues and infertility in women.

Gallstones

Gallstones are hard pieces of stone-like material that form in the gallbladder. They're mostly made of cholesterol. Gallstones can cause stomach or back pain.

People who are overweight or obese are at increased risk of having gallstones. Also, being overweight may result in an enlarged gallbladder that doesn't work well.

Many of these deadly diseases are not just a theory for me, they have actually impacted my life and altered it dramatically.

Yep, there it is, obesity can lead to Congestive Heart Failure. Oh and Congestive Heart Failure can lead to early death. I say that with indisputable authority. Oh look obesity can also lead to High Blood Pressure. Yep, that at least temporarily grounded me as a pilot. Oh and by golly obesity can also greatly increase your chances of getting Type II diabetes. Yeah, I proved that true also. And then there is abnormal blood fats also known as high cholesterol. I got that too. And now the grand prize, obesity also aids and abets cancer. Well at least I did not get menstrual issues. Clearly obesity is far more than a mere personal fashion statement. It may not in and of itself be specifically a deadly disease but it sure helps a lot of deadly diseases advance within our bodies. But just in case you don't quite get it yet let's look at what some of the obesity generated or obesity aggravate diseases can do to you beyond just dying.

Type II diabetes seems relatively innocuous. Yeah okay so maybe you have to spend the rest of your life jabbing yourself with a needle every day, maybe a few times every day, just to give your body needed insulin. But what else can happen, especially if you ignore your new diet requirements and/or your insulin injections It can get really ugly.

Complications from Type II diabetes includes increased opportunity for heart and blood vessel diseases such as coronary artery disease, heart attack, stroke and even more opportunity for high blood pressure. You will also almost always get some degree of neuropathy or more simply nerve damage. That can lead to all sorts of nasty things up to and including the development of gangrene requiring amputation. There is also increased likelihood of kidney damage, eye damage, foot damage, hearing impairment and even Alzheimer's disease. Remember this all goes back to obesity. How does that box of donuts sound now?

And then there is that lovely and very deadly disease, Congestive Heart Failure. This is not a heart attack, although obesity increases the risk of heart attack as well, but Congestive Heart Failure is its very own very nasty disease. Essentially what happens with CHF is that the heart weakens and it becomes increasingly difficult for it to effectively pump your blood to where it is needed around your body. At first the heart may just stretch to hold more blood but eventually the heart weakens leading to the kidneys responding by causing the body to retain fluids. That can cause fluid to build up in your arms and legs, feet and perhaps most dangerously in your lungs. That is what actually took me down. You see when your lungs fill with fluid you just cannot breathe and the inability to breathe will quickly kill you. It is all related to obesity. Do you still want to super-size those fries? Really?

As they say in those always fun to watch infomercials on TV, "But wait there is more." Let us not forget high blood pressure also known as hypertension. Some of the highlights of the many joys (he said sarcastically) of high blood pressure is the increased opportunity for artery damage, aneurysm, coronary artery disease, enlarged left ventricle (heart), stroke, dementia and kidney failure. So what do you think should we run out and get another six pack? This is all related to obesity folks, there is a lot more than just being "pleasantly plump" and letting our belts out a notch or two. This is something that left ignored can kill you or render you far more ill than you ever imagined. And now the grand prize, obesity contributes to cancer.

Let me emphasize something very important here. When you read these words, "Diabetes, Coronary Heart Disease" and even "Cancer" the all too human reaction is to think vaguely that yes these are terrible diseases but heck I won't get THAT. Even more deluding is that for darn near everyone there is no real understanding of just how awful and painful any of these conditions can be. You don't just get cancer and drop dead. The same is true for any disease mentioned here. What actually happens is that things fall apart relatively slowly but steadily making your life a living hell until it ends. Here is just one tiny example.

I knew a guy once who had become enormous, well in to the realm of severe obesity. His doctors told him that he really needed to lose weight, to which he responded by ignoring the problem. Then one fine day the doctors told him that he had achieved the acquisition of Type II Diabetes. Congratulations! He was given blood test

strips and a prescription for insulin. He did use both
more or less but he steadfastly refused to alter his diet.

Consequently one day he noticed a dark sort of bluish
greenish spot on his left foot so he went see his doctor.
It turned out that the spot was gangrene and to hopefully
stop it from spreading they had to amputate his left leg at
the knee. This is absolutely one of the consequences that
can flow from Diabetes. But my friend still saw no good
reason to alter his diet so about two years later he lost his
other leg. Eventually he lost both legs and both arms
and finally it completely consumed him and he finally
died a very painful and miserable death. For virtually
everyone a story like that while tragic is nevertheless
about some other person and it can never happen to me,
right? Wrong! Smart people learn from their mistakes,
if they survive them but even smarter people learn from
the mistakes of others.

Now that you have this information you must take that
always crucial first step and fully own the problem. It is
YOU, no one else. YOU are obese and being obese is
not just unpleasant it can lead to early and painful death.
Obesity goes way beyond a simple fashion statement,
left ignored it can truly kill you. Know this, own this
and the solutions will rapidly become available to you.
Yes, doing this can be uncomfortable at first but once
you grab a hold of the problem the light begins to shine
through because then and only then will you see the path
out of obesity hell.

Far too often what people try to do is find a quick and easy solution to this seemingly overwhelming problem. Sure there are surgical techniques that might be beneficial but frankly I don't think so. I mean seriously think about it. First you have to go under a general anesthesia which is in and of itself something that is loaded with danger and risk. Then someone cuts open your skin and then goes on to hack away at the fat tissue to remove it from your body. This procedure, no matter how professionally done, cannot help but to bring trauma to your body and leave behind significant scar tissue. And then there is the cost in dollars. But, of course, if you think such surgery is what you want by all means do confer with your physician for serious medical advice. And I will add that in those rare circumstances of wildly extreme obesity that we hear about on the news from time to time, cases such as a thousand pound man or woman who have to be extracted by a crane and transported on a truck bed; those people may truly have no option but surgical assistance as a desperate attempt to literally save their life. But those are extreme and rare cases. For most of us basically eating less and better while increasing physical activity will resolve the problem.

Yet some of us will shun the surgical approach but will instead gravitate towards a vast variety of quick weight loss programs that involve things such as "cleanses" or the ingestion of various herbs and other "natural" elements that claim to dramatically aid in reducing weight.

In my opinion none of this necessary or beneficial. Now that you have truly taken full ownership of the problem the very best solution is right there in your hands. What you must do is make critical lifestyle changes. You can evolve into those changes over time, just not too much time. And typically the required changes are not wildly radical and not at all painful. Best of all perhaps is that you can do this without attacking your body with a sharp instrument or draining your bank account.

Now that we clearly and undeniably know that obesity is your problem let's move forward with how you can resolve it – permanently.

Celebrity Moment One

To illustrate just how powerfully deadly obesity can be, how it can literally kill even the rich and famous I will now take pause for a celebrity moment. Here then is my first celebrity.

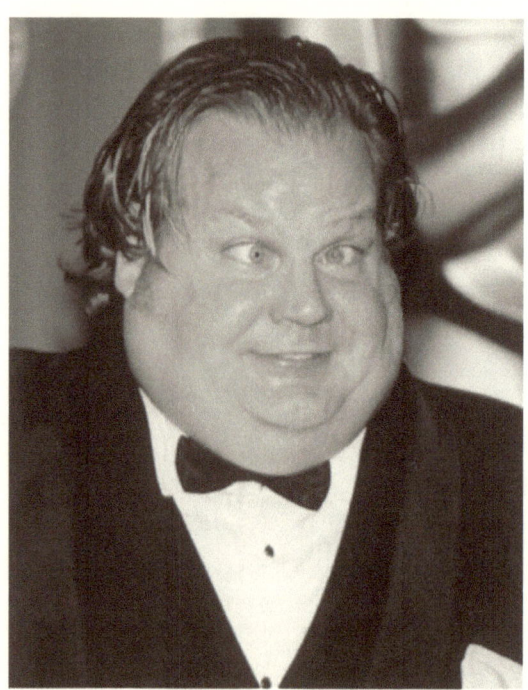

You remember this guy, right? It's **Chris Farley**. Born in Madison, Wisconsin on February 15, 1964 he quickly rose to a position of fame when in 1990 he joined Saturday Night Live and soon formed an alliance with Chris Rock, Adam Sandler Ron Schneider and David Spade. He also had prominent roles in feature films *Wayne's World, Coneheads, Airheads, Tommy Boy* and *Black Sheep*. By any rational measure Chris Farley was a show business success story. His personal life, however was in many ways a total wreck leading to his untimely death at the tender age of only 33. The official cause of death was deemed to be a drug overdose, but the autopsy also revealed that Chris Farley suffered from advanced atherosclerosis which was cited as a "significant contributing factor" in his demise.   That condition was directly related to Chris Farley's obvious extreme obesity.

This is in a no way a put down or slams Chris Farley. What it is and the only purpose it serves is to clearly illustrate how universal and deadly obesity truly can be. No amount of fame of fortune will protect a person from the ravages of obesity. It also demonstrates clearly just how difficult dealing with obesity can be. I will never know, of course, but I would be willing to bet that had Chris Farley been able to obtain this book and follow its guidance there is a good chance he would still be alive entertaining the world.

Eat Less and Move More

Well that is basically the solution so I guess the book ends here. Okay there is more to consider and I will get to that but at the core is the need to eat less and move more. Way too many of us have allowed ourselves over time to get sedentary while at the same time satisfying ourselves by consuming abundantly all of those foods that make us feel good and bring us at least temporary joy but often long term disaster.

There was once a time when the sedentary element was reserved primarily for stressed out adults whose work requirements stole their energy and desire for more physical activity. The youngsters were typically fine as they would get out of school and go play vigorously and engage in a wide range of physical activities. But to far too great an extent those days are now ancient history. The internet, smart phones, text messaging and all manner of the burgeoning digital world have brought far too many of our youth to a near standstill. Pushing on the smart phone is not even close to the energy level and calorie burn of more old school activities such as playing softball or basketball or just plain running and walking around. To be sure those activities do still exist but for far too many of our modern youth life has become far too sedentary. Unfortunately the typical nature of youthful eating habits hasn't changed much if at all. Kids still love those milkshakes and who wouldn't love a great big juicy double cheese burger with a super-sized order of French fries? The result is that childhood obesity has become a huge epidemic in America and around much of the world.

Regardless of your political position I do fully support Michele Obama's efforts to get American youth to move more. Just how effective her campaign turns out to be at least a powerful woman in the position of being First Lady has taken a stance and that is one much needed step towards overall better health for our population.

That still leaves the adult population and that group seems to be sinking ever deeper into the hole of despair and obesity. Yes I said "despair" because to a very significant extent there is a link between depression and other negative mental conditions and obesity. For one heck of a lot of us one solution when feeling down is to grab something wonderful and jam it down our throats. A little sad, grab a couple of doughnuts. Feeling a little blue, there isn't anything quite as nice as a great big slice of banana cream pie with two scoops of our favorites ice cream to make us happy again. Then, of course, there is the biggest potential threat to our overall health, the use of alcohol to rid ourselves of those bad days and lousy memories. That can and often does lead to a wide variety of disasters on many levels.

Along with the all too often disastrous dietary choices we indulge ourselves in, there is the concurrent condition of ever shrinking physical activity. Darn near every American adult owns an automobile. Perhaps in major urban environments such as New York City maybe not, but there instead the good people extensively rely upon public transportation to reduce to near zero actual walking.   In my own particular case for far too long I would always take the car to go a mere half mile to the local grocery store. The mere thought of actually walking that half mile, about 1000 steps was simply unthinkable.

Even in our homes darn near everything these days can be controlled by a remote; our televisions, our radios, even our lights are often dealt with by a simple push of a button. There is no need to actually stand up and walk over to a device to change it; just press a button. So we sit in our easy chairs with the remote in one hand and our smart phones in the other as our derrières get ever larger. This near total lack of any meaningful level of physical activity doesn't apply to everyone, of course, but it applies far more so than it once did. But as bad as lack of physical activity is, it is the food we consume that can really do us in.

In his book *Dr. Neal Barnard's Program for Reversing Diabetes* Dr. Barnard tells a little story of a man he and a colleague Dr. Stanley Talpers, MD met one day at the George Washington University School of Medicine in Washington, DC. The patient had not been losing weight and offered the opinion that what he needed to do was to walk more. Dr. Talpers then vigorously recommended that the patient concentrate much more on modifying his diet because according to Dr. Talpers to lose one pound walking you would need to walk from Washington, DC to Baltimore, Maryland a distance of approximately 38.5 miles. The point here is a simple but critical one and that is making essential modifications to your diet is an absolute must if you are to win the battle with obesity. And yes, getting good and sufficient exercise is also important, but proper diet is far more important to weight control. And by the way, I highly recommend Dr. Neal Barnard's book for while it is focused on diabetes, diabetes and obesity often go hand in hand and much of the material in his book is solid information on how to construct a healthy diet based on real science.

So it is absolutely correct to say that to achieve a much better level of health one needs to eat less and move more but that doesn't tell the whole story. It is not only how much we eat but what we eat that makes the biggest difference in our overall health. With that said let's move on to the most critical element in our overall health, our diet. It is absolutely NOT A DIET but our diet that matters most.

Celebrity Moment Two

To illustrate just how powerfully deadly obesity can be, how it can literally kill even the rich and famous I will now take pause for a celebrity moment. Here then is my second celebrity.

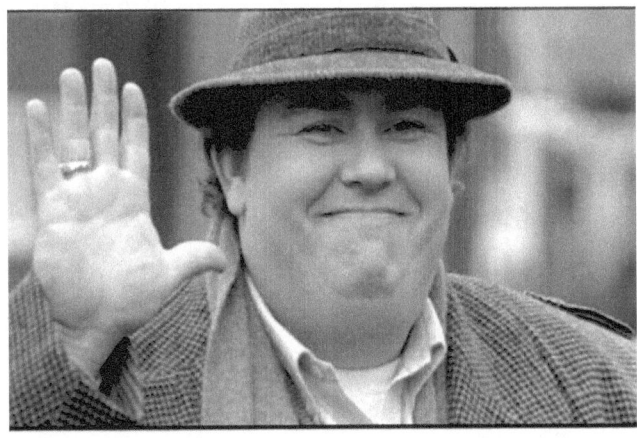

John Candy was a brilliant comedic actor born October 31st 1960 in Newmarket, Ontario, Canada. John Candy honed his craft as a member of the Toronto branch of *Second City*. He was a major player on *Second City Television* and appeared in many movies including Stripes, *Splash, Cool Runnings, Summer Rental, The Great Outdoors, Spaceballs* and *Sumer Rental* to name but a few. It is fair to say that as the performance career of John Candy developed he truly became a rich and famous man and he was absolutely a man of enormous talent who often played characters that were both funny and loveable.

But sadly John Candy died on March 4th 1994 only 43 years old. He should have had decades more to practice his craft and entertain his legion of fans but he was struck down by a heart attack, yet another condition which may or may not have been caused by obesity but in any event is always exacerbated by obesity.

No disrespect to John Candy but I have to also mention just how ironic it is that his name was "Candy" and one of his very last films was "*Canadian Bacon.*" Coincidence or prophetic, you decide. Either way it was yet again a tragic and almost assuredly preventable loss of a life.

Good Food Bad Food

What needs to be fully understood is that there are foods that are good for you health wise and foods that are absolutely bad for you health wise. A big problem arises when the bad food tastes great and the good foods are boring. Happily there is a solution but first let me identify some basic bad foods and some basic good foods.

First let's look at some general rules. Basically if it grows out of the ground and doesn't contain a deadly poison it is good for you. Also as a generally rule if it is an animal product it should either be avoided altogether or consumed in extreme moderation. Also add to the list of substances to be avoided are these three components found in food. Sugar, salt and fat. In fact one of the most powerful tools I used during my period of major weight reduction was this little graphic that I placed prominently on my refrigerator door. You might want to do the same thing.

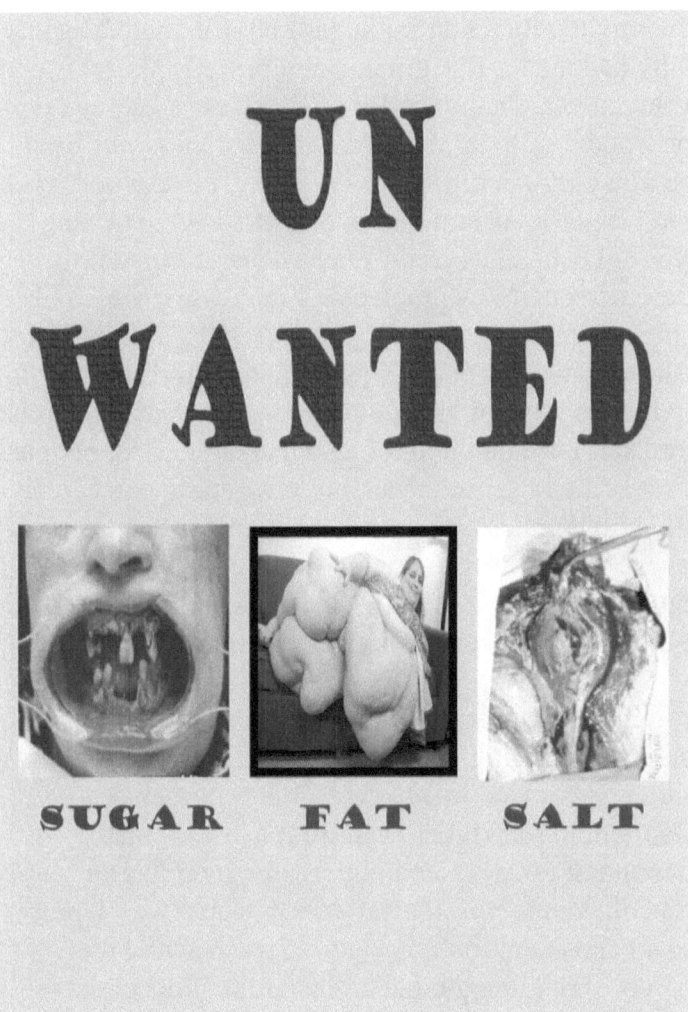

You might notice that for sugar I have a photo of some really bad teeth. It is graphic and powerful but it is not by any means the totality of what excess sugar can do to you r body. Too much sugar also damages your liver and you only get one of those. It also raises your A1C or blood sugar level and that in turn can lead to getting Type II Diabetes. For fat I used a photo of a wildly obese person. Now granted as I said eating well and achieving and maintaining proper healthy weight is not a fashion statement but this particular photo is so over the top it does send an undeniable message. Finally for the word salt I used a photo of an aneurysm. Most people never actually see an aneurysm but getting one can be fatal. So the message conveyed by this little poster is I believe rather powerful and it does serve as a great reminder of some of the most significant things to avoid or at the very least significantly minimize in our diets.

Also in the category of things best left off your plate would be anything deep fat fried and especially when as it often is covered in a batter. This is particularly important to remember because it is not all that uncommon to take something really good like say broccoli, smother it in a batter and deep fry it. Upon casual consideration it is a good food because it is broccoli. But the good qualities of the broccoli have been overrun by the strong negatives of the batter and the deep frying. It is an easy trap to fall into.

Also basically all processed meats should be strictly stricken from your personal menu. I mean really who doesn't just love a few big slices of a nice salami or summer sausage both of which contain wildly excessive amounts of sodium and fat. Two of the three "Unwanteds" and since they also frequently also contain a surprising level of sugar as well you can get all three of the "Unwanteds" in just one somewhat tasty food.

Meat in general is not in the most favored category and there are plenty of people including vegetarians and vegans who will tell you that all meat is just plain bad. Maybe but in my world an occasional and modest serving of chicken or turkey without the skin or a piece pork with the fat trimmed off or a lean piece of beef will find its way to my dining table. The key here is to keep it small and infrequent. It also allows for a fair enjoyment of key holidays such as Thanksgiving. In other words you don't have to become a total food snob or social outcast to eat healthy. What you must do, however, is take complete control over your personal menu and severely moderate certain foods such as meat products.

Another area where near total rejection is appropriate is any form of ice cream, pies, cakes and candies. All of the above are saturated in sugar and sugar is actually addicting. Feeding a sugar addiction never has a good result. And other then the candies these foods also typically contain significant levels of fat thereby by hitting two out of three of the "Unwanteds."

Now sure you can be polite and accept say ONE piece of chocolate at the office party unless, of course, you know damn well that taking one piece will quickly lead to a second and third and fourth and then oh what the hell you lost count. That such a possibility exists suggests that at least at first your best course of action is to politely decline any offer of any of these foods and candies.

Also smarten up and learn to always read the BACK label of every food item you may want to consume. Food marketers are very smart and they know well the buzz words that will ensnare you. Have you ever seen, for example, a package of something with a bold statement such as ORGANIC,: ALL NATURAL or LOWER FAT and GLUTEN FREE and you immediately think well heck this is something healthy. Well it could be but it also may well not be. Pick up the package of whatever it is that has your interest and read fully the nutritional details printed on the back or maybe on the side of the package. You will be enlightened and probably shocked. Sugar, fat and salt are all natural and for that matter so is arsenic. But the back label may well disclose that the "ALL NATURAL" product you are looking at has massive quantities of one or more of the "UNWANTEDS." As for that LOWER FAT claim the first question I ask is, yeah lower than what? Again the nutritional information will disclose just how much fat the product contains. To be sure some fat is not just okay but even desirable However the general rule is a maximum of 70 grams of total fat and not more than 24 grams of saturated fat per adult per day. Personally I strive for something below half those numbers but never ever exceed those numbers.

As for the latest crazy of gluten free, that really only matters if you happen to be one of the very very few people with a gluten allergy. If that is you then, of course, by all means avoid the gluten but for the overwhelming majority of people gluten is of no particular consequence.

The bottom line on this topic is that to concentrate on what essentially is mere marketing ploys emphasizing gluten free, non GMO and organic while ignoring the far more meaningful issues of sugar, fat and sodium content is the equivalent of picking at gnats while swallowing elephants. Sure it can all matter but for your basic health it is nutritional realties that matter most.

While discussing daily amounts of things we can consume in our diets for salt the maximum amount is 2300 milligrams and for sugar the maximum amount of daily consumption is just 90 grams. Again I much prefer an amount of about half of these numbers, but under no circumstance do you ever want to exceed these amounts. However, how can you know what your consumption is if you don't invest a tiny amount of time checking the actual nutritional information for all of the foods you eat? The obvious answer is that you just can't so guess what now your grocery shopping has become just a wee bit more time consuming. But hey, that's okay because by eating smart and right you will have a whole lot more quality time on earth.

Now let's look at some of the very best foods we can eat. Here is a short list:

Black Beans	Kale
Salmon*	Walnuts
Pumpkin	Apples
Blueberries	Banana
Broccoli	Spinach
Sweet Potatoes	Kidney Beans
Celery	Carrots
Lentils	Red Beats
Brussels Sprouts	Steel Cut Oatmeal
Bulgur	Flaxseed
Chia Seeds	Almonds
Tuna*	Fat Free Yogurt
Green Onions	Peaches
Pears	Cabbage
Lettuce	Mushrooms

By way of a good general guide if it grows out of the ground it is good. But do notice I included both salmon and tuna. They are both excellent sources of Omega 3 fatty acids but caution, in the case of both salmon and tuna the preference should always be for wild caught fresh fish and never the canned variety. Also baking is preferred to frying but if you absolutely must fry I would suggest the use of Buttered Flavored Cooking Spray which has zero everything accept flavor.

You also need to exercise your brain a little when considering foods such as pumpkin or even apples. The basic food is fine but using that fact to justify a great big slice of pumpkin or apple pie topped with whipped cream and a side of ice cream is absolutely not the correct approach. Similarly indeed steel cut oatmeal is a good food but not when covered with brown sugar, butter and cream. Got it? This may seem like a simple idea to grasp but often it isn't all that simple because we all love to play games with ourselves when we really want to keep feeding our bad diet habits. So yes I am afraid that if losing weight and then maintaining good healthy weight is your goal it is absolutely essential to pump up your discipline.

My Diet Choices Then and Now

Now let's add some real world experience to this discussion. I will start with an example of what my personal food consumption was like as I rose all the way up to the staggering weight of 315 pounds. Then I will provide you with a real world example of what my typical daily diet is now that I am at 165 pounds with every intent of remaining there or maybe slowly losing even a couple of more pounds. To give this even more meaning I am a male 5 feet 10 inches tall. Here goes.

In those wild old days....

	Cal	Fat	Sodium
Breakfast:			
Two eggs fried	164	14g	188mg
Hash browns	470	31g	746mg
4 strips of bacon	166	13g	543mg
2 pieces rye toast	166	2g	422mg
A bowl of fruit	70	0	15mg
1 glass of 2% milk	130	5g	120mg

	Cal	Fat	Sodium
Lunch:			
Half pound burger	840	50g	1510mg
French fries	582	28g	625mg
1 slice carrot cake.	246	12g	233mg

Diner:

	Cal	Fat	Sodium
1 vanilla milkshake	560	26g	272mg
1/2 roasted chicken	1890	30g	3720mg
Mash Potato +gravy	230	5g	780mg
Peas	134	1g	382mg

DAILY TOTALS	5648	217g	9556mg

So on a very typical day during my fat man period I sucked into my body an outrageous 240% of the maximum calories recommended for my age weight, height and activity level, a phenomenal 297% of the recommended maximum daily intake of total fat and a mind blowing 398% of the maximum allowance of sodium intake. And I didn't even include the butter I used in making some these foods and I never considered myself a particularly heavy eater. Oh and to be sure I had a snack or two at night typical washed down with a glass of wine. In hindsight it seems a miracle that I am still alive and able to share this information with you. Remember at this time my weight fluctuated between a low of around 260 pounds to an all-time peak of 315 pounds. Even at my low end I was roughly 100 pounds above ideal weight and my health was indeed rapidly deteriorating.

Oddly I felt fine. Oh to be sure I couldn't walk very far and certainly not up very many stairs or on an up sloping terrain before becoming winded, but hey just don't walk up long stairways or hills and everything was simply fine. But in truth I was coming apart fast on my inside. My blood pressure was beginning to rage; heck with a daily sodium intake of an amazing 9556mg of sodium a day I am surprised by veins didn't just explode. Another happy by product of all that sodium was significant fluid buildup throughout my body. That led to nicely swollen arms and legs and feet, a condition that went mostly unnoticed. It was also a byproduct to the Congestive Heart Failure that was lurking within me. But what the hell those darn big burgers at Wendy's and Fuddruckers are spectacular and who doesn't like a great big delicious milk shake, right?

Ah an then totally unnoticed by the more or less conscious me was what was happening to my liver. It seems bombarding your body with outrageous amounts of sugar, fat and salt plays havoc with your liver and that it often shows up as that magnificent disease known as Type II Diabetes.

Meanwhile I just kept chowing down enjoying every morsel. Sure I realized that I had become "a bit" over weight – A BIT! So every once and awhile I would cut back a little and I would also try one of those miracle supplements to hasten the shedding of my excess weight. But it was clearly a case of too little too late. So one fine day my lungs filled with fluid, I could not breath and the heart dropped to zero function. That friends is called death. Due to far more extremely good luck than I deserved my big fat dumb ass was saved by an extremely competent EMT Team. After 26 days in the hospital even I came to understand that it was long beyond the time I took my health seriously and so a new approach was clearly needed.

So once I decided to do everything I could to shed the wildly excessive weight and hopefully return to far better level of health here is what my typical daily diet had evolved into.

	Cal	Fat	Sodium
Breakfast			
Two soft boiled eggs	136	9g	244mg
1 slice Flaxseed bread	50	1g	60mg
One banana	105	1g	1mg
Lunch			
1 Cup broccoli	50	1g	49mg
1 Cup Cauliflower	28	0g	9mg
¼ Cup pasta	75	1g	3mg
¼ Cup pasta sauce	80	1g	300mg
1 veggie burger	120	4g	398mg
Dinner			
1 cup mixed vegetables	120	1g	64mg
4 oz. white chicken meat	141	3g	99mg
1 slice flaxseed bread	50	1g	60mg
½ cantaloupe	95	1g	44mg

DAILY TOTALS	1050	24g	1331mg

Now that is a monster change and much healthier. And yes I know you are thinking, "but dude that is such tasteless boring food." Well you are absolutely wrong but I understand your thoughts because when you like me are in the habit of wolfing down massive amounts of fat and sodium and sugar and calorie rich foods it is easy to form the opinion that foods with much less of those elements must be bland and boring. Happily once you actually try foods similar to those given above you will find as I did that that they can be very satisfying. There are, however, a few tricks to improve the taste and enjoy ability.

For example in my fairly typical lunch meal I will sprinkle just a wee bit of crushed red pepper on the food. Just a little bit is all you need but it will absolutely spark up the taste. Also not included above but often consumed by me are blueberries. I grant you that just plain blueberries are somewhat dull, but add a little almond milk and sprinkle them with a wee bit of Stevia and viola' you have a truly delightful eating experience.

Also please understand that while I try to be as precise as possible with the numbers sited for each food element it is impossible outside of a laboratory environment to be absolutely precise. I mean did you serve yourself exactly one cup of whatever or could it have been 1.1 cups or 1.2 cups or maybe just .9 cups? But these variances are not particularly important so long as you do make an effort to be honest with yourself.

Also you must be willing to experiment with a variety of foods. As you do experiment always keep in you're mind the three major "Unwanteds" and you should be just fine. The overall goal is to significantly reduce your consumption of fats, particularly saturated fats, sodium a/k/a salt and the big kahuna CALORIES. The somewhat over simplified but nonetheless valid general rule is "Burn more calories than you consume and you WILL LOSE WEIGHT."

Think of it as if you were a very unique hybrid automobile. Your gas tank holds precisely one gallon and only one gallon. One gallon of gas will carry you exactly 20 miles. At the end of the twentieth mile your vehicle will run out gas and it would stop except for its one unique feature. Overtime your unique car absorbs a substance I will call gas-fat. It is held in various locations around the car body and may even cause the car to have lumps here and there. But as you reach the twentieth mile your car can no longer fuel itself from the gas tank so it begins to draw from the gas-fat. Keep driving and eventually even the gas-fat will be exhausted but all of those lumps will also be gone. That is in a very simplified but essentially correct description of how your body handles calories and accumulated fat. When you exhaust the currently available calories the body draws from the accumulated fat and happily you will lose weight.

Now many books on this topic will include extensive meal menus. I am not going to do that for many reasons. One is that I am lazy, but the far more noble reason is that if you are going to modify your behavior successfully you will need to learn how to determine your own foods and not simply depend on someone else's concepts. What I have offered here is a basic prototype from which you can build your own healthy meals. Just always keep in your mind the need to minimize FAT, SUGAR and SALT you will be well on your way to far healthier eating and living. To accomplish that means also that from this day forward you will invest some time at the grocery store looking not only at the front labels designed exquisitely by the marketing department, but far more importantly at the back labels where the real nutritional information reposes.

Yet another great source as you begin to build your healthier meals is this web link. http://nutritiondata.self.com/. There you will find an extensive data base of all of the nutritional elements for the vast majority of food stuffs on our planet.

When shopping for food you can largely ignore all of those ever more popular claims such as: organic, gluten free, GMO free, reduced fat and other claims that are for the most part are more a matter of marketing than any real health significance. I will grant you that in some foods the organic claim has real merit and if you are one in the many millions who do suffer from a gluten allergy then, of course, you should avoid gluten. But the always important elements to consider are the levels of calories, sodium, fat and sugar present in each and every food item you might consume. Essentially all of that information is available right on the label. But obviously in things such as fresh vegetables and fruits you will need to look elsewhere for that information and for that you need merely to go the website given above.

I offer one final admonishment before moving on to the area of moving more also known as exercise. Transition gradually but steadily. People who go wildly off in a desperate attempt to trim down fast by switching from over easting of mostly not so good foods to grossly under eating of any kind of food will ALWAYS 100% of the time snap back in short order and regain roughly 120% of whatever weight they might lose in their frenzied efforts. Take it easy but steady. Set goals one week at a time. Take off say 10% of your total calorie consumption each week until you reach your optimum level. **Give your body and mind time to adjust because what this must be about is a lifestyle change that is real and permanent and not yet another quick fix.**

Thanks to the internet age we live in there is one awesome tool available absolutely free that can help you every step of the way and it is called *MyFitnessPal* and you will find it right here: https://www.myfitnesspal.com/. It is a extremely helpful site that will help you set and attain rational goals. It offers detailed analysis of pretty close to every imaginably food on earth. It is a snap to set up and extremely easy to use. Just go to the sight and follow the simple directions. You set up your individual site by entering essential data such as your age, weight, height and gender. Then you have options in establishing your weight lose goals. Again I recommend that you start slowly and increase your loss rate as you grow more comfortable with the modifications you make. I used it extensively and still use it to keep on track. In addition to its abundant reservoir of critical information about every imaginable food by using it every single time you put something in your mouth and swallow it you are doing the one thing that will ultimately allow you to take full control of your own health and well-being and that one things is DISCIPLINE. Probably for the very first time in your life you will be actually thinking about every single thing you eat and that is the only way you can truly take full control. It is a beautiful thing. Now let's do as Taylor Swift says and let's Shake it Off.

Celebrity Moment Three

To illustrate just how powerfully deadly obesity can be, how it can literally kill even the rich and famous I will now take pause for a celebrity moment. Here then is my third celebrity

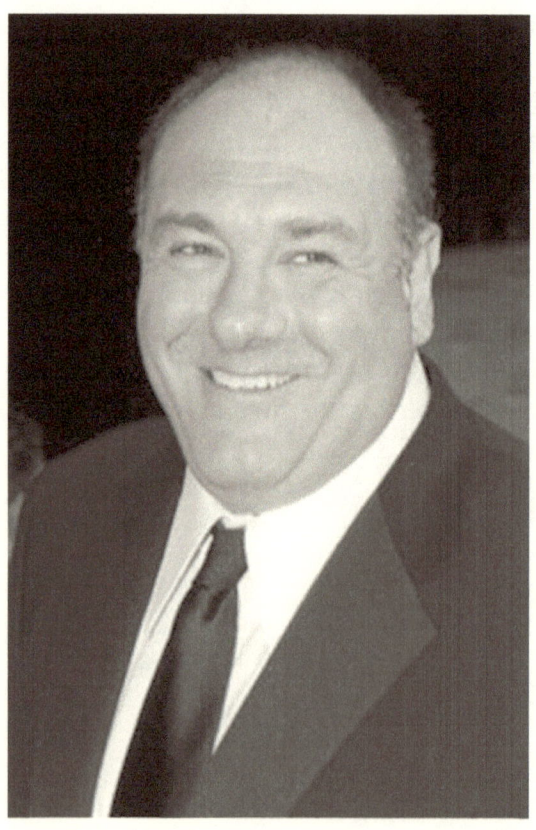

James Gandolfini was born in Westwood, New Jersey on September 18th 1961. He didn't begin his acting career until he was in his twenties but it didn't take James Gandolfini long to prove his star qualities. By 1992 he arrived on Broadway playing alongside of Jessica Lange and Alec Baldwin in a revival of *A Street Car Named Desire*. His break out movie was as a hit man in Tony Scott's 1993 film *True Romance*. However it was his portrayal of mob boss Tony Soprano in the smash hit television series *The Sopranos* that elevated James Gandolfini to true star level.

But fame and fortune were not enough to give James Gandolfini a long life because while on vacation in Rome, Italy James Gandolfini was stricken with a massive heart attack or more precisely cardiac arrest and that ended his life at the all too young age of just 41 years.

Yet again the ravages of obesity conquered another supremely successful mega star. I will say that I was one of his fans and I thoroughly enjoyed each and every one of his performances in *The Sopranos*. His sad and early death brought pain and sorrow to millions. The good news, the only good news is that maybe the tragic lose of yet another major celebrity might be useful in helping others still living to take the steps needed right now to reshape and rebuild our own lifestyles in such a way that we might enjoy much longer and happier lives.

May you rest in peace James Gandolfini.

Move It

I said it before and I will say it again, when it comes to weight loss diet is 80% of the equation and exercise is but 20% but that 20% is absolutely vital for many reasons. For one thing one law of physics certainly applies and that is that a body at rest tends to stay at rest. The less egghead version of that is if you have fallen into the trap of mostly sitting on your butt that is most likely what you will continue to do right up until you just keel over and fade to black. Our bodies are designed to move and when that movement stops or diminishes significantly the body begins to rebel internally. Blood pressures tends to rise, fat tends to more aggressively accumulate with the very severe risk of clogging arteries. Muscles can atrophy and by the way, you do recall from high school biology that the heart is a muscle. Plus try hard to remember the first ten years or so of your life. Odds are you will recall that you were exceedingly active. There are exceptions, of course, but by natural design we are born to move. Heck even before birth our little developing children start kicking their way into our world. Movement is natural and right, absence of movement is potentially deadly.

However, I once again say that what needs to be done is to gradually but steadily begin to increase your activities. Attempting to go from devoted couch potato to Olympic athlete runs a very serious risk of untimely death as you shock your system dramatically. Also this would be a good time to again suggest strongly that before getting into any significant exercise program you pay a visit to your physician and get a full review of your true physical condition. Tell your physician what your plans are and heed his or her advice. Then start slowly and build up your activities gradually. Here are couple of examples.

Let's say that you are now motivated to get back in the game so to speak. You recall that when you were younger you really enjoyed playing tennis. You were never anywhere near the super star level but you could and did get the ball over the net and in the court regularly and most of all you enjoyed doing it and so now you want to do that once again. But unfortunately you have put on 60 extra pounds and you haven't done much more physically over the last several years beyond walking to the refrigerator to grab another beer. So by all means do pick up that tennis rack, stop by the sporting goods store and grab a few new tennis balls and head off to the court. But start nice and slow. If available perhaps begin by banging a few balls off of a wall, or maybe rent a ball machine to toss a few at you. You will quickly discover that you now suck at tennis but not to worry. Your first time back on the court limit yourself to no more than say 30 minutes and do NOT push yourself very hard. But do go back every second or third day. Eventually you will see and feel a difference in your performance and gradually you can increase your time on the court from 30 to 40 and then 60 minutes. Each step along the way you will feel new energy fill your body and that will be a truly glorious feeling. Never really cared much for tennis, fair enough.

Go look in your garage and perhaps you will find that nice bicycle you once rode extensively. Oops! It seems covered with cobwebs, and look there are rust spot here and there. No problem, just take it to the bike shop and in a day or two it will be almost as good as new for a tiny fraction of what new bike would cost. So the bike will be good again but odds are not you. So again start slow, maybe just one mile on day one. Perhaps give yourself a schedule of a ride every other day increasing the distance and/or time by say 20% on each successive outing. Eventually you will begin to feel totally at ease and confortable back in the saddle and that is exactly what your goal should be. But there is life beyond bicycles.

Depending on where you live swimming can also be a fantastic way to reenergize your body. Here, where I live in Southern, California swimming is not a very difficult task, but in Bent Fork, North Dakota it might be a bit challenging. Whatever your circumstance may be it is yet again imperative that you start slow BUT stay on it regularly gradually increasing your efforts over a reasonable amount of time.

Our world is now also abundant in gyms. Going to the gym can be a great way to reawaken long ignored muscles and rebuild your tired old body. Most gyms also have the benefit of one or more trained men or women known as trainers who can help you put together a program that can maximize your gains from the gym experience. Both the gyms and the trainers do cost, however, so you will have to factor that into your total approach as well. One could say something like "well my health has no budget" but that can be a tad optimistic in the real world. You are the only person who can ultimately make that decision. It would be rather counterproductive if you begin reviving your physical health only to suffer from the stress of spending beyond your actual means. But there is one physical activity that I personally have come to love and it costs absolutely nothing.

Walking is a great exercise on many levels. It is NOT particular aerobic, however, you can interject periods of jogging in your walks thereby adding an aerobic element. Some people do better when they engage in exercise with other people and some people prefer being alone. Walking allows for both options. There are walking clubs in many communities where you can join with others for a nice healthy walk. How much you walk is as always a very individual matter and as with all exercise you must start slow especially if you have been sedentary for a long time.

When I first started to get back into walking I was happy if I walked one lousy mile a day. For me that was a walk to a nearby grocery store and back. But once I started walking I gave up my frankly stupid habit of always driving to that store even if only to pick up one or two items. What a total waste of gasoline. Now, unless I am going on a major shopping spree I walk to the store every day often several times a day. But well beyond the grocery store I now walk all over my home town and have in process not only greatly improved my fundamental health but have also rediscovered my absolutely beautiful hometown. Yes, of course, I started slow, but now I walk no less than 10 miles every single day and I do so at pace that varies between 4.5 and 3.5 miles per hour. Within my first 30 minutes the endorphins start to kick in and I begin to feel a natural high far better than anything any drug could possibly induce. I can leave my home grumpy but I am ALWAYS happy when I return. This is one great way to rejuvenate body, mind and soul.

But I don't stop there. I also have developed a routine of other exercises. For me it includes various forms of calisthenics to help limber up and a few weight exercises just to tone my puny muscles. But these routines are purely personal and you will likely find various elements that particularly suit you. The important key is first and foremost DO IT. But that said, start slow and grow at a steady but rational pace. Always get good medical advice before launching into any significant exercise routine. And you may well settle in on one preferred kind of exercise and that is fine so long as you do supplement it with other activities so that you are benefiting your entire body and not only one muscle group. There is absolutely no reason for your exercising to be uncomfortable or painful when implemented properly. In fact what you should discover is a brand new sense of tremendous comfort and joy throughout your body and within your mind. This rapidly becomes something you really love to do and no longer something someone else tells you that you have to do.

NOTICE please that nowhere in this discussion did I make firm statements about specific exercises. There is no benefit in me or anyone else telling you that you MUST do 100 jumping jacks, 50 push-ups and run three miles before breakfast every day, The exact nature and extent of your exercising must be of your choosing if it is to become what it must become and that is your whole new lifestyle. To be sure gaining knowledge and getting some guidance along the way is helpful, but in the end it is your life and your lifestyle that matters. Just be sure that you focus on a lifestyle that is centered on genuine health because that will bring you happiness at level you probably never before even imagined.

East Conquers West

There has long been much discussion about the intriguing consequences of East meeting West. But in one instance it has clearly become a case of East in a way conquering West. How so you ask? From mostly unknown obscurity only a few decades ago Yoga has swept the Western world and with it has come significant benefit.

Yoga began in ancient India centuries before the birth of Christ. Yoga is a practice that combines the body the mind and the spirit of its devotees. There are a variety of different "schools" of Yoga but as their particular approaches vary the essential essence remains the same.

Today Yoga schools are almost as popular throughout the Western World as fast food restaurants – almost. However, yoga has far more benefit to offer. At its core yoga is a method employed to achieve liberation. Its actual practices do vary depending upon which particular theology and philosophy you may follow but central to all is that it provides a disciplined method for attaining a goal. Yoga offers techniques for mastering your body and mind. But at its core yoga is a Hindu based practice that has grown over many centuries and has become highly popular in the Western world as a form of conditioning of both body and mind. You will almost certainly think of yoga primarily as a number of "positions" the adherents assume. This is how it is typically presented in the modern Western world. However its roots are far richer and deeper than what is typically offered at your local gym. Nevertheless yoga has many benefits and is well worth your consideration as yet another tool that can be effectively employed to help you attain your personal goals of health and balance in life. So while yoga may or may not be something you will embrace on your path to building a new and healthier lifestyle, it at the very least deserves a look.

For a more detailed and comprehensive overview of the ancient and venerable practice of yoga you may want spend a little time at this website: https://en.wikipedia.org/wiki/Yoga.

Celebrity Moment Four

This time we have a relatively rare WINNER! This celebrity began her public performing career noticeably larger than good health would dictate. However in her case she shed the weight while building her career. Here then is my fourth celebrity moment. Take a look at this.

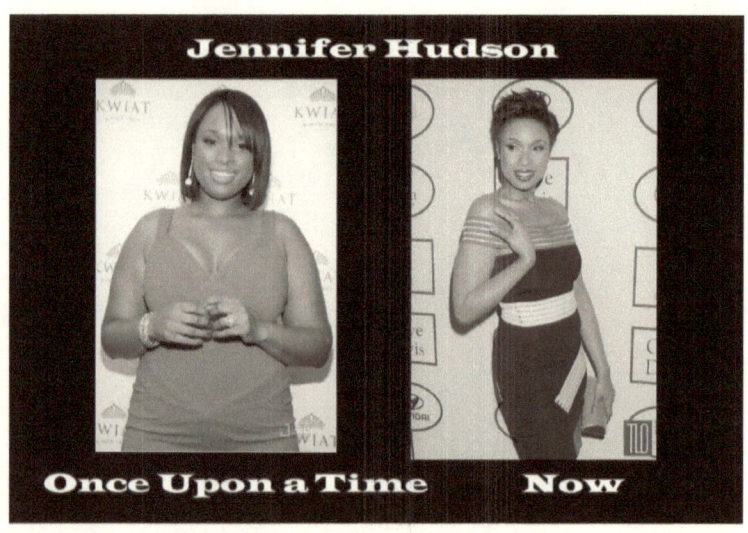

And our WINNER is none other than the dazzling Jennifer Hudson. A beautiful and multi-talented Chicago girl Jennifer Hudson leaped into national fame when she competed on American Idol. Her talent was clear and she soon became signed to a major record label. Beyond that Jennifer Hudson soon found herself cast in the film adaptation of *Dreamgirls* where she worked with super stars Jamie Foxx, Beyonce Knowles and Eddie Murphy. She has accumulated an amazing number of awards for her efforts and remains a still rapidly rising star. She is also a clear and positive example of the reality that you really can beat obesity. Congratulations Jennifer Hudson.

Twists and Turns

As you embark on this whole new and wonderful lifestyle expect and be prepared for some indeed many twists and turns, failures and setbacks. That is to be expected and it is perfectly natural and it absolutely does not mean that YOU are a failure in any way. Yes, of course, there will be frustrations and disappointments. There will be times when after what you believed was a great week of self-control on your *MyFitnessPal* program only to step on the scale and watch it go above the previous week by a pound or two. There will be days when despite your very best efforts you just won't have the energy to drag yourself out to the gym, or the tennis court or any other physical activity you had planned. Sometimes a setback of that sort may be as the result of some infirmity like a cold or other routine malady of man. And sometimes it will just be a reaction to the changes you are bringing upon yourself. At times your mind and body just won't focus in the way you intended. Occasionally the results you so enthusiastically anticipated just won't show up. Expect these moments and accept them as a natural and normal party of your growth and development. After all it is certain that it took a long, often a very long time to get yourself into bad shape so you cannot realistically expect to turn it all around in a week or a month of even several months What you will be embarking on is a lifelong adventure with no absolute destination and no firm time schedule. It is all about changing the process and as you succeed one step at a time positive results will take care of themselves. Accept this reality and make but one promise to yourself. Promise that you will simply never ever quite your pursuit of a better, stronger, healthier and yes happier life. Keep that promise to yourself and it will happen.

One sure way to experience quick failure is to overdo it out of the gate. For years you have steadily slipped into a condition that you have finally decided to get yourself out of. That is great news and so you read this book and set out to achieve your goal. Your goal is to lose 20 or 40 or 60 pounds and to do as fast as you possibly can. So you use *MyFitnessPal* but you start off setting your target at 1000 calories a day. Then to further enhance your condition you go to a gym and sign up for several high intensity classes from day one. Such action guarantees failure for several reasons. First of all again you must understand fully that what you want to accomplish is a long term lifestyle change and not a quick fix. Put yourself on a starvation diet and you may well lose weight for a week or two or three, but sooner or later and most likely sooner you will snap and snap hard. You conclude that you are on an impossible mission and its killing you so you will dive deeply back into the bad old habits. Disgusted with your enormous discomfort at being in a state of starvation you will react by wildly over indulging in every bad food at a mind blowing and truly gut busting level. Or you will find that the sudden huge burst in physical activity is not just difficult it is downright painful so you will just flat out quit.

Much of this can be avoided by starting off gently and gradually increasing your efforts on both of the major fronts. That is start by aiming for just one half pound per week in weight loss. And keep your physical activity at a level that is comfortable to you increasing it gradually over time. To be sure, especially with an aggressive trainer you will be pushed to maximize your efforts. That's okay but never to the extent where it pushes you right out of the door and back to the lounge chair. It is a lifestyle change, something that must and will literally stay with you for the rest of your life so with very rare exception there is no sense of urgency other than the understanding to start TODAY. Start today yes, but you cannot and will not and there is absolutely no need to attempt to get it all done today or tomorrow or next week because again I say – this a process, a journey and not a destination.

So when you hit a bump, when you do get temporarily side tracked, just pick yourself back up and get back in the game. There is no need to feel guilty or angry or sad. So long as you stay on that train or having fallen off get right back on that train to better health and happiness the destinations will over time take care of themselves. Disappointments, expect them and simply commit yourself to never ever under any circumstances just quit. It is an inalienable truth that quitters don't win and winners don't quit.

With food you should experiment. Always keep in mind to minimize your intake of fat, sugar and salt, but reach way beyond this modest text and search an ever increasing variety of conforming options to enjoy. Basically every fruit and every vegetable is on the good list and even those foods that are marginal or even on the do not eat list may be consumed occasionally in small amounts. And yes you can give yourself an occasional cheat day. Set aside two days each month when the rules can be suspended and you can join me in that delicious carrot cake or that New York Strip steak, only now you will order the 6 ounce steak rather than the 12 ounce and you will enjoy it immensely.

Be suspicious of the never ending flood of gimmicks. It is impossible to go through most grocery store checkout counters without seeing magazines with headlines screaming such claims as "New Miracle Food Lose 30 Pounds FAST." Maybe, I really doubt it but maybe it will actually perform as claimed but nevertheless so I promise you that even it did work as advertised you would lose 20 pounds this month and get 30 pounds back next month because once again it is not consistent with a life style change but yet another bogus quick fix. Over time you will begin see these ads for what they are, bogus gimmicks that entrap the unaware. But with each day you work at shaping your new lifestyle such gimmicks will become less and less of interest to you as your full understanding of the real world continuously expands.

In the realm of physical fitness there are another whole set of traps and dangers. Once again it is a matter of moving steadily and positively but at a pace reasonable for you. A particular trainer may well push you far harder than you find comfortable. Talk with him or her but if you cannot reach an accord walk away. Also really think about what you are doing. I joined a gym and found myself mainly using the treadmill and the weights. But then I came to understand that if I merely walked to the gym and back I would have more exercise than I would get from the treadmill and I have a fairly substantial collection of weights at home, so what was the point. But that is me. Many people find a degree of support surrounding themselves with others striving for great fitness. I fully understand that desire and it makes a gym membership a truly valuable tool for many. So my argument is neither join a gym or don't join a gym or hire a trainer or don't hire a trainer, but rather know why you want the gym membership and hire only such trainer who is actually working with you in helping you to achieve your goals, not his.

How to Handle Eating Out

It is often a pleasant interlude in our lives, to dine out with friends, family and a special someone. Other times it is basically a necessity. You are out and about taking care of life's details and you need to grab a bite to eat. Either way to stay on top of your game you will need to have some idea of the nutritional aspects of your restaurant meal. Interestingly most major fast food chains such as McDonald's and Subway make nutritional information about their various foods readily available. Many restaurants are putting at least the calorie content of their various food items known to the consumer, but rarely is the complete nutritional break down including elements such as sugar, sodium and fat made known. Sometimes your *MyFitnessPal* will provide you with a decent guestimate but sometimes not. So what do you do?

Basically I would recommend that you try to limit your restaurant experience to those establishments that do make the nutritional components of their food readily known to its customers. However, when that fails and *MyFitnessPal* strikes out you should treat that incident as one of your "cheat days" and enjoy the dining experience.

Even with compromise you do, however, need to exercise some common sense. Clearly, for example, avoid the obviously over the top selections.

As you begin to build your new, stronger and healthier life here are a few observations that can help make the process a little more successful. Outback Steakhouse for example has a dish they call "Bloomin' Onion." It is essentially a gigantic deep fried onion and holds a staggering 1954 calories, 155g of fat, 18g of sugar and a heart killing 3841mg of sodium. But in fairness that is for the entire product. They claim each "Bloomin Onion" equals a total of six servings. So when you divide those numbers by six the amount per serving isn't all that damaging. But this is the kind of information you will need to keep yourself on the right track.

Other menu items to avoid even when exact nutritional data is not available is anything deep fried, smothered in butter or cream sauce or covered with a crispy crust. Of course, there are also those very tempting desserts. A mere half cup of a typical chocolate mousse for example brings 454 calories, 77g of sodium, 32g of fat and 30g of sugar to your body. Seems like a lot of "Unwanteds" for a mere half cup.

While many restaurants still don't make the nutritional informational available on their menus you can often get that information from their website before you go. So when you are planning a social or family meal out, take the couple of minutes necessary to get a full run down and what is involved. Plan your meal wisely and then execute your plan.

In general mostly avoid restaurants where nutritional information is not available but if you can't avoid such a restaurant for whatever reason, use your common sense and minimize your portions and save such days as one of your limited cheat days.

Some Tricks and Tips

Always, always and always keep in your conscious mind the fact that what you are doing is reconstructing your fundamental lifestyle. Always take that approach and never ever allow yourself to think that you are on some sort of diet. Yes, you must and you will modify your dietary intake but that is not the same as going on a diet. A few other things you can do to strengthen this process is to always give yourself a little bit less than you might at first desire. Be sure to consume sufficient water and avoid virtually all carbonate beverages "diet" or otherwise. The water will actually help remove or reduce the feeling of hunger making taking in less food just that much easier. When you employ this technique throughout the day every day it will soon become a routine and very positive habit. Your new motto will become "Less is Better."

One thing I found that is extraordinarily helpful in building and strengthening my self-discipline was to very consciously consider many of the bad foods and beverages that I once so thoroughly indulged myself with. For example, I would go to the bakery department of one of my favorite food stores and I would look long and hard at let's say an great big beautiful carrot cake. As I stared at the cake I would consciously force myself to contemplate the deep displeasure of having to jab myself with a needle so as to inject insulin into my body because my previously dietary habits had wreaked havoc upon my liver and I had to deal with the ravages of Type II diabetes. As I stood there staring I would see another person, clearly obese walk by and put a pie or box of cookies or other "goodies" into his or her shopping cart and I would remind myself of just how easy it would be to fall back down that hole. It never took very long before my mind firmly shifted to a solid commitment to totally and cheerfully avoid what I had once thought of as a true treasure. True health won the moment.

Yes I know this is fairly hardcore and not everyone will want to copy it, but it has worked very well for me. Psychologists would I believe call this a form of adverse conditioning. For me it works and it works well.

Ironically this seems to have worked so well that now when I allow myself to indulge in some of these once favored but clearly undesirable foods, I don't like them very much anymore. This applies to all manner of super sweet pastries, cakes, cookies and pies as well as such once upon a time delights as hamburgers and even steak. On those now extremely rare moments when I allow myself to eat such things I find that they no longer appeal to me all that much. Apparently my new lifestyle transformation has worked very well and yours can as well.

Of course there are still times during the day when I need a little food pick me up. Only now rather than grabbing a candy bar or a donut I grab a handful of grapes or an apple of maybe a pear. I also make darn sure to enter that food into *MyFitnessPal*. I ingest far less calories, fat, sodium and sugar than was previously the case and yet I really am still satisfied.

Also on the matter of movement, force yourself to do more. Even little things can, over time, add up to make a big difference. For instance don't always fight for the parking space closest to the door. Rather, intentionally and willingly park across the lot where there are plenty of open spaces and you will be able to walk a little more getting in and out of the store or office you are visiting. Doing this may seem somewhat counter intuitive at first but that will change over time and you will not only be getting a wee bit more good exercise you will also be cutting down on the stress inherent in always trying to get the parking spot nearest the entrance. More exercise and less stress, a perfect combination.

In a somewhat similar vein begin using stairs rather than an elevator when you are only going up five levels or less. It is a great add on to your overall exercise and its absolutely free. There are no gym fees required but it absolutely helps in your overall commitment to moving more.

Also whatever you do AVOID those devices that do indeed help to lose weight but solely by causing you to sweat profusely thereby dumping water weight, but only water weight and with the very dangerous opportunity for dehydration.

Last but absolutely not least there is the matter of clothing and of particular importance shoes. Whether in the gym or the great outdoors it is essential that you dress to the circumstances. What does that mean? It means keeping your clothing lite on the hot days and warm on the cool days and generally avoid extreme weather. It also means to wear protective clothing appropriate to the activity. Men do need some good protection of their private parts in sports activates that put their sensitive areas at risk. Women need to take somewhat similar measures with respect to their breasts. It would be abhorrent if you were to suffer a major or possibly even life threatening injury while attempting to improve your overall health. There are, of course, nearly endless varieties of physical activities and not only sports. Each activity has its own inherent risks and there is always at least some protection provided by wearing the clothing and protective gear appropriate to the circumstances.

Of great importance, particularly if you are to embark upon substantial walking, jogging, running of hiking is proper footwear. This is one area in which you should absolutely not cut corners. Really good running and walking shoes will cost around $150.00 and they are worth every cent both in terms of comfort and protection for your feet and legs. You might get lucky and pay a little less or you may see something extraordinary and pay a bit more but if you think paying $150.00 for good shoes is expensive just wait until you get your medical bills for treating all of the injuries that can occur from having inappropriate or poor quality footwear. But deciding on exactly what appropriate foot wear is required is something you must do for yourself with some guidance from some good sporting goods store employees. In some areas of our country there are stores that specialize in foot wear. If such a store exists in your area I would recommend that you pay them a visit. Getting the right foot wear will greatly improve your comfort and your safety and that will contribute generously to your overall success and happiness. No really, shoes matter.

Water

The amount of water in the human body ranges from 50-75%. The average adult human body is 50-65% water, averaging around 57-60%. The percentage of water in infants is much higher, typically around 75-78% water, dropping to 65% by one year of age. Consequently whenever we discuss things such as weight loss, exercise and even overall lifestyle changes some attention must be given to water in a broad sense and hydration in a slightly more narrow sense. Following is an excellent overview of the whole issue of dehydration from the good people at the Mayo Clinic. Do please pay close attention as it can be a deadly mistake.

Dehydration occurs when you use or lose more fluid than you take in, and your body doesn't have enough water and other fluids to carry out its normal functions. If you don't replace lost fluids, you will get dehydrated.

Common causes of dehydration include vigorous exercise, especially in hot weather; intense diarrhea; vomiting; fever or excessive sweating. Not drinking enough water during exercise or in hot weather even if you're not exercising also may cause dehydration. Anyone may become dehydrated, but young children, older adults and people with chronic illnesses are most at risk.

You can usually reverse mild to moderate dehydration by drinking more fluids, but severe dehydration needs immediate medical treatment. The safest approach is preventing dehydration in the first place. Keep an eye on how much fluid you lose during hot weather, illness or exercise, and drink enough liquids to replace what you've lost.

Mild to moderate dehydration is likely to cause:

Dry, sticky mouth

Sleepiness or tiredness — children are likely to be less active than usual

Thirst

Decreased urine output

No wet diapers for three hours for infants

Few or no tears when crying

Dry skin

Headache

Constipation

Dizziness or lightheadedness

Severe dehydration, a medical emergency, can cause:

Extreme thirst

Extreme fussiness or sleepiness in infants and children; irritability and confusion in adults

Very dry mouth, skin and mucous membranes

Little or no urination — any urine that is produced will be darker than normal

Sunken eyes

Shriveled and dry skin that lacks elasticity and doesn't "bounce back" when pinched into a fold

In infants, sunken fontanels — the soft spots on the top of a baby's head

Low blood pressure

Rapid heartbeat

Rapid breathing

No tears when crying

Fever

In the most serious cases, delirium or unconsciousness

Unfortunately, thirst isn't always a reliable gauge of the body's need for water, especially in children and older adults. A better indicator is the color of your urine: Clear or light-colored urine means you're well hydrated, whereas a dark yellow or amber color usually signals dehydration.

When to see a doctor

If you're a healthy adult, you can usually treat mild to moderate dehydration by drinking more fluids, such as water or a sports drink (Gatorade, Powerade, others). Get immediate medical care if you develop severe signs and symptoms such as extreme thirst, a lack of urination, shriveled skin, dizziness and confusion.

Treat children and older adults with greater caution. Call your family doctor right away if your loved one:

Develops severe diarrhea, with or without vomiting or fever

Has bloody or black stool

Has had moderate diarrhea for 24 hours or more

Can't keep down fluids

Is irritable or disoriented and much sleepier or less active than usual

Has any of the signs or symptoms of mild or moderate dehydration

Go to the nearest hospital emergency room or call 911 or your emergency medical number if you think a child or older adult is severely dehydrated. You can help prevent dehydration from becoming severe by carefully monitoring someone who is sick and giving fluids, such as an oral rehydration solution (CeraLyte, Pedialyte, others), at the first sign of diarrhea, vomiting or fever and by encouraging children to drink plenty of water before, during and after exercise.

Dehydration occurs when there isn't enough water to replace what's lost throughout the day. Your system literally dries out. Sometimes dehydration occurs for simple reasons: You don't drink enough because you're sick or busy, or because you lack access to safe drinking water when you're traveling, hiking or camping.

Other dehydration causes include:

Diarrhea, vomiting. Severe, acute diarrhea — that is, diarrhea that comes on suddenly and violently — can cause a tremendous loss of water and electrolytes in a short amount of time. If you have vomiting along with diarrhea, you lose even more fluids and minerals. Children and infants are especially at risk. Diarrhea may be caused by a bacterial or viral infection, food sensitivity, a reaction to medications or a bowel disorder.

Fever. In general, the higher your fever, the more dehydrated you may become. If you have a fever in addition to diarrhea and vomiting, you lose even more fluids.

Excessive sweating. You lose water when you sweat. If you do vigorous activity and don't replace fluids as you go along, you can become dehydrated. Hot, humid weather increases the amount you sweat and the amount of fluid you lose. But you can also become dehydrated in winter if you don't replace lost fluids. Preteens and teens who participate in sports may be especially susceptible, both because of their body weight, which is generally lower than that of adults, and because they may not be experienced enough to know the warning signs of dehydration.

Increased urination. This may be due to undiagnosed or uncontrolled diabetes. Certain medications, such as diuretics and some blood pressure medications, also can lead to dehydration, generally because they cause you to urinate or perspire more than normal. So once again we see the far reach inherent in obesity associated diseases including diabetes which in turn can cause a vast array of other troubling medical and health problems including

dehydration. Obesity truly is the gift that keeps on giving; you just don't want t=what it has to offer.

Anyone can become dehydrated if they lose too many fluids. But certain people are at greater risk, including:

Infants and children. Infants and children are especially vulnerable because of their relatively small body weights and high turnover of water and electrolytes. They're also the group most likely to experience diarrhea.

Older adults. As you age, you become more susceptible to dehydration for several reasons: Your body's ability to conserve water is reduced, your thirst sense becomes less acute, and you're less able to respond to changes in temperature. What's more, older adults, especially people in nursing homes or living alone, tend to eat less than younger people do and sometimes may forget to eat or drink altogether. Disability or neglect also may prevent them from being well nourished. These problems are compounded by chronic illnesses such as diabetes, dementia, and by the use of certain medications.

People with chronic illnesses. Having uncontrolled or untreated **diabetes puts you at high risk of dehydration.** But other chronic illnesses, such as kidney disease and heart failure, also make you more likely to become dehydrated. Even having a cold or sore throat makes you more susceptible to dehydration because you're less likely to feel like eating or drinking when you're sick. A fever increases dehydration even more.

Endurance athletes. Anyone who exercises can become dehydrated, especially in hot, humid conditions or at high altitudes. But athletes who train for and participate in ultramarathons, triathlons, mountain climbing expeditions and cycling tournaments are at particularly high risk. That's because the longer you exercise, the more difficult it is to stay hydrated. During exercise, your body may lose more water than it can absorb. With every hour you exercise, your fluid debt increases. Dehydration is also cumulative over a period of days, which means you can become dehydrated with even a moderate exercise routine if you don't drink enough to replace what you lose on a daily basis.

People living at high altitudes. Living, working and exercising at high altitudes (generally defined as above 8,200 feet, or about 2,500 meters) can cause a number of health problems. One is dehydration, which commonly occurs when your body tries to adjust to high elevations through increased urination and more rapid breathing — the faster you breathe to maintain adequate oxygen levels in your blood, the more water vapor you exhale.

People working or exercising outside in hot, humid weather. When it's hot and humid, your risk of dehydration and heat illness increases. That's because when the air is humid, sweat can't evaporate and cool you as quickly as it normally does, and this can lead to an increased body temperature and the need for more fluids.

Dehydration can lead to serious complications, including:

Heat injury. If you don't drink enough fluids when you're exercising vigorously and perspiring heavily, you may end up with a heat injury, ranging in severity from mild heat cramps to heat exhaustion or potentially life-threatening heatstroke.

Swelling of the brain (cerebral edema). Sometimes, when you're getting fluids again after being dehydrated, the body tries to pull too much water back into your cells. This can cause some cells to swell and rupture. The consequences are especially grave when brain cells are affected.

Seizures. Electrolytes — such as potassium and sodium — help carry electrical signals from cell to cell. If your electrolytes are out of balance, the normal electrical messages can become mixed up, which can lead to involuntary muscle contractions and sometimes to a loss of consciousness.

Low blood volume shock (hypovolemic shock). This is one of the most serious, and sometimes life-threatening, complications of dehydration. It occurs when low blood volume causes a drop in blood pressure and a drop in the amount of oxygen in your body.

Kidney failure. This potentially life-threatening problem occurs when your kidneys are no longer able to remove excess fluids and waste from your blood.

Coma and death. When not treated promptly and appropriately, severe dehydration can be fatal.

So is there any doubt about just how important hydration and the truly critical role water play in our basic survival? But that raises another interesting category of concern and that is, what about the quality of the water we drink?

The sad truth is that water from municipal water systems is often subpar. Here is just one of many stories about poor municipal water. This one appeared in Daily Finance and was written by Douglas McIntyre.

Unknown to most Americans, a surprising number of U.S. cities have drinking water with unhealthy levels of chemicals and contaminants. In fact, some organizations and state environmental agencies that collect and analyze water data say the level of chemicals in some Americans' drinking water not only exceeds recommended health guideline but the pollutants even exceed the limits set by the U.S. Environmental Protection Agency (EPA), the national legal authority in these matters.

The website 24/7 Wall St. examined the quality of water supplies in most major America cities, using data collected from multiple sources for five years (ending in 2009) by Environmental Working Group (EWG), based in Washington, D.C. The fact that the data covered a half-decade is important because it shows that the presence of certain chemicals is persistent.

Cities in Kansas, Louisiana, Mississippi, Tennessee and Georgia provided insufficient data to be included in EWG's database. Some other major cities outside of these states also failed to submit information, including Detroit, Salt Lake City and Washington, D.C.

Test results from EWG's national database covered "a total of 316 contaminants in water supplied to 256 million Americans in 48,000 communities in 45 states." According to the data, among the contaminants were 202 chemicals that aren't subject to any government regulation or safety standards for drinking water.

Based on the EWG's methodology, 24/7 Wall St. came up with its 10 worst cities list. These cities' water quality rank is based on three metrics, in order of increasing importance:

The percentage of chemicals found based on the number that were tested for

The total number of contaminants found

The most dangerous average level of a single pollutant.

Here's that list, in descending order, with the city's water utility in parenthesis:

10. Jacksonville, Fla. (JEA)

Located on the northeast coast of Florida, Jacksonville is the state's largest city. According to EWG, 23 different toxic chemicals were found in Jacksonville's water supply. The chemicals most frequently discovered in high volumes were trihalomethanes, which consist of four different cleaning byproducts -- one of which is chloroform. Many trihalomethanes are believed to be carcinogenic. Over the five-year testing period, unsafe levels of trihalomethanes were detected during each of the 32 months of testing, and levels deemed illegal by the EPA were detected in 12 of those months. During at least one testing period, trihalomethane levels were measured at nearly twice the EPA legal limit. Chemicals like arsenic and lead were also detected at levels exceeding health guidelines.

9. San Diego (San Diego Water Department)

Located on the Pacific in Southern California, San Diego is the country's eighth-largest city. According to California's Department of Public Health, San Diego's drinking water system contained eight chemicals exceeding health guidelines as well as two chemicals that exceeded the EPA's legal limit. In total, 20 contaminants have been found. One of those in excess of the EPA limit was trihalomethanes. The other was manganese, a natural element that's a byproduct of industrial manufacturing and can be poisonous to humans.

8. North Las Vegas (City of North Las Vegas Utilities Department)

North Las Vegas's water supply mostly comes from groundwater and the Colorado River, and doesn't contain chemicals exceeding legal limits. However, the water supply did contain 11 chemicals that exceeded health guidelines set by federal and state health agencies. The national average for chemicals found in cities' water exceeding health guidelines is four. North Las Vegas had a total of 26 contaminants, compared with the national average of eight. The water contained an extremely high level of uranium, a radioactive element.

7. Omaha (Metropolitan Utilities District)

The land-locked city of Omaha gets its water from the Missouri and Platte Rivers, as well as from groundwater.

Of the 148 chemicals tested for in Omaha, 42 were detected in some amount, 20 of which were above health guidelines, and four of those were detected in illegal amounts. These were atrazine, trihalomethanes, nitrate and nitrite, and manganese. Atrazine is an herbicide that has been shown to cause birth defects. Nitrate is found in fertilizer, and nitrite is used for curing meat. Manganese was detected at 40 times the legal limit during one month of testing.

6. Houston (City of Houston Public Works)

Houston is the fourth-largest U.S. city. It gets its water from sources such as the Trinity River, the San Jacinto Rivers and Lake Houston. Texas conducted 22,083 water quality tests between 2004 and 2007 on Houston's water supply, and found 18 chemicals that exceeded federal and state health guidelines, compared to the national average of four. Three chemicals exceeded EPA legal health standards, against the national average of 0.5 chemicals. A total of 46 pollutants were detected, compared to the national average of eight. The city water has contained illegal levels of alpha particles, a form of radiation. Similarly, haloacetic acids, from various disinfection byproducts, have been detected.

5. Reno (Truckee Meadows Water Authority)

(UPDATE, April 29, 2014): DailyFinance was recently contacted by representatives of the Truckee Meadows

Water Authority, which strongly disputes the accuracy of the EWG report upon which this article was based. To quote their email:

"The data that was used originally to rank some of these utilities is wrong, namely TMWA. ... One of the many errors: the data they used was for RAW water, not finished water that people drink. ... We contacted EWG and they agreed to correct the data and re-rank us. ... It never happened.

Their full public response to the alleged errors can be found here. We have contacted the EWG for comment. When they reply, we will let our readers know. In the meantime, however, with no revised data to go by, we cannot update this listing. So, read on, but with the caveat that the Reno data is contested.)

Reno gets most of its water from the Truckee River, which flows from Lake Tahoe. Of the 126 chemicals tested for in Reno over four years, 21 were discovered in the city's water supply, eight of which were detected in levels above EPA health guidelines, and three of these occurred in illegal amounts. These were manganese, tetrachloroethylene and arsenic. Tetrachloroethylene is a fluid used for dry cleaning and as an industrial solvent, and is deemed a likely carcinogenic by the International Agency for Research on Cancer. Arsenic is a byproduct of herbicides and pesticides, and is extremely poisonous to humans. During at least one month of testing, arsenic levels were detected at roughly two and a half times the legal limit.

4. Riverside County, Calif. (Eastern Municipal Water District)

Riverside county is a 7,200-square-mile area located north of San Diego, part of California's "Inland Empire." The county is primarily located in desert territory, and so the water utilities draw their supply from the Bay Delta, which is miles to the north. The water in Riverside County contained 13 chemicals that exceeded recommended health guidelines over the four tested years, and one that exceeded legal limits. In total, 22 chemicals were detected in the district's water supply. The contaminant exceeding legal health standards was tetrachloroethylene.

3. Las Vegas (Las Vegas Valley Water District)

Located in the Mojave desert, Las Vegas gets its water from the Colorado River through miles-long intake pipes. While its water doesn't exceed the legal limits for any single type of contaminant, Las Vegas's water has a large range of pollutants. Of the 125 chemicals tested for over a five-year period, 30 were identified in some amount, and 12 were found in levels that exceeded EPA health guidelines. These chemicals included radium-226, radium-228, arsenic and lead. The two radium isotopes are commonly found around uranium deposits and are hazardous to human health, even in small quantities.

2. Riverside, Calif. (City of Riverside Public Utilities)

Riverside, with a population slightly greater than 300,000, gets most of its drinking supply from groundwater. Regulators in the city of Riverside, which has a different water-treatment facility than the rest of Riverside County, detected 15 chemicals that exceeded health guidelines and one that exceeded legal standards. In total, 30 chemicals were found. Since 2004, the water has almost consistently been riddled with alpha particle activity, traces of bromoform (a form of trihalomethane) and uranium, causing an unusually unhealthy water supply.

1. Pensacola, Fla. (Emerald Coast Water Utility)

Located on the Florida Panhandle along the Gulf of Mexico, Pensacola is Florida's westernmost major city. Analysts say it has the worst water quality in the country. Of the 101 chemicals tested for over five years, 45 were discovered. Of them, 21 were discovered in unhealthy amounts. The worst of these were radium-228 and -228, trichloroethylene, tetrachloroethylene, alpha particles, benzine and lead. Pensacola's water was also found to contain cyanide and chloroform. The combination of these chemicals makes Pensacola's water supply America's most unhealthy.

So with all of these rather scary stories what do people do? What people often do is buy and consume bottled water. But consider this. Often times bottled water is no better than and sometimes even worse than the municipal water supply. So now where do you go. Water is clearly one of our most critical resources, but how do we get in good clean safe form?

For years now there has been an industry devoted to providing effective water filters. Like all human creations some work better than others. But for well over two decades now I have been using a Multi Pure drinking water filter and it has proven to be extremely effective, simple and easy to use and vastly less expensive than bottled water. If you happen to have an interest in the product check them out at: http://www.multipure.com/. But then there is the next level.

It has been postulated that ionized water and reducing its acidity yields a superior water. One of the leaders in this field is Kangen Water. You can get a good overview of their products and the science behind what they do by starting at this website: http://www.enagic.com/watertheory.php.

There has been a growing legion of people who claim that their use of Kangen water has dramatically changed their lives for the better. That might seem ridiculous at

first blush, but when you fully grasp just how critical water is to human life it becomes much more plausible. I was also impressed by a special report on a local CBS TV Los Angeles. Here is that report.
https://www.youtube.com/watch?v=Twx8YKFhZRs

What, if any of these issues at least intrigue you? Given the undeniable significance of water these issues should grab your attention; so by all means do take the time to check it all out. The one statement I will make is that if you are concerned about your tap water do use a high quality filter. Also, when it comes to hydration it is all about good, purified clean straight up water. Sugary carbonated drinks should be kept to an absolute minimum.

BS. Lots of large people live long and well.

I can hear your voices all over the world. Many of you are saying: "Oh come on Dude, there are plenty of plus sized people who live long and happy. Heck my granddaddy was over 300 pounds and drank like a fish. He lived to 98, so your whole premise is just plain BS."

Heck I will even admit to something that is very similar in nature. Way back in 1981 and 1982 my life was in turmoil and I found myself consuming copious amounts of alcohol. Worse than that, much worse I also frequently drove a car while significantly under the influence of that alcohol. I am certainly not proud of that dark spot in my personal history but I never once got arrested for DUI nor did I ever once have a car crash while under the influence of alcohol. So does that support the notion that drinking and driving is a good thing?

Here is an even stronger argument. Sir Winston Churchill successfully led his nation, England through and out of the hell known as World War Two. Surely he was under extreme stress on a daily basis. Perhaps as result of that stress or maybe just because of a particular aspect of his personality Sir Winston Churchill was also known to smoke cigars frequently and consume significant amounts of cognac every day. He was obviously a portly man well within the arena of obese. Yet despite all of these things Sir Winston Churchill lived to the ripe old age of 89. Indeed it was Sir Winston Churchill whom I regular cited in my frequent denials of my own obesity.

It is so darn easy, isn't it? I mean truly there are so many examples of people who break the rules and live seemingly well beyond what one might expect giving their wild and crazy lifestyles. But does that mean we should copy those lifestyles? And yes it is true some day we will indeed all die, so what is the issue here? Why not live life to the maximum and not worry about some silly ass health issues that may or may even touch us?

Well let me start with a few other observations.

One of the more interesting things I participated in as a young Marine was executing a field of interlocking fire at night using tracer rounds. The reason it was at night and tracer rounds were employed was to vividly demonstrate just how devastating such a field of fire truly can be. I mean what we saw appeared to be impenetrable. There was simply no way in hell anyone could walk, run or crawl through such a field of fire and live. Yet in actual combat many people indeed traverse similar fields of fire and lived to tell about it.

I also once met a man who claimed, and I believed him, was a pilot in the Israeli Air Force. Not just once but on two separate occasions he was forced to eject from his aircraft. In both instances his parachute failed to deploy. Yet he obviously had survived not just one but two instances of departing an aircraft in flight and surviving the experience without a parachute. So does that mean you should go out and join a sky diving club and practice jumping out of an airplane without a chute? Hey why not, one guy did essentially that and lived to tell about it.

Indeed our world is replete with many examples of people who have lived on the edge and sometimes well over the edge and yet survive. So is that really a good argument for our own poor behavior and lack of good judgment?

And as for the well we will all die anyhow argument as convincing as that may seem on the surface it misses one huge point and that is not just the quantity of life but the quality of life. Okay so no matter how we live someday we will die, so let's just live wild and crazy and enjoy it all. That might work, but you are really fighting against enormous odds. And one ugly surprise you put yourself at risk for is a situation where you don't just die, but rather you find yourself wrapped in a miserable painful disease that torments you every day and night.

So sure why not just for fun go out and get into a wrestling match with a hungry lion. The lion will simply eat you and its over in a flash. But get and remain obese and among a huge menu of ugly options you may well get Type II Diabetes and Type II Diabetes can easily lead you into that dark place where gangrene infects your body and then you face a series of amputations and an ultimately painful death. THAT is one of the big differences. Not only length of life but quality of life.

The more you ignore the realities the more likely you are to spend a very long time in misery and pain. It is in the end all about the odds for as you have correctly surmised there is no such thing as a sure thing except for eventual death.

So until that final day comes wouldn't it be wise to do all that you can to live a truly happy, healthy and mostly pain free life? And by the way having personally been on both sides of this story I can tell you that without exception my overall joy of living is far greater now having embraced a far healthier lifestyle. My energy level is close to what it was in my twenties, my joy of life has never been stronger and I am so deeply happy to be able to enjoy my beloved family and many friends every single healthy day. Heck since starting on this far healthier path I have had precisely ONE day of severe cold symptoms over a period approaching three years.

ONE day of sickness in three years is a pretty good record I think.

So the real BS element here is in continuing to use those well-known exceptions in a vain attempt to ignore the basic reality. Sure you might survive and you might live to be 100 and you might even enjoy most of that time in outwardly decent health, but attempting to do is wildly playing a major long shot.

The one thing you need to remember from all of this is that unfortunately should you eventually come to understand the far greater wisdom of dedicating your life to solid good health is vastly better than ignoring the risks and living a wild and reckless life is that by the time you come to understand the true depth of you error it will almost certainly be far too late to do much about it.

Stevia

There is something new and seemingly miraculous that is sweeping the modern industrialized world. It is a sweetener that is all natural and literally hundreds of times sweeter than sugar, but contains no sugar and no chemicals. We call it Stevia. Lovers of sweetness rejoice.

Stevia is perhaps unique among food ingredients because it's most valued for what it doesn't do. It doesn't add calories. Unlike other sugar substitutes, stevia is derived from a plant.

The stevia plant is part of the Asteraceae family, related to the daisy and ragweed. Several stevia species called "candyleaf" are native to New Mexico, Arizona and Texas.

But the prized species, *Stevia rebaudiana* (Bertoni), grows in Paraguay and Brazil, where people have used leaves from the stevia bush to sweeten food for hundreds of years. In traditional medicine⬈ in these regions, stevia also served as a treatment for burns, colic, stomach problems and sometimes as a contraceptive.

Today, stevia is a big and growing part of the sugar substitute market.

The U.S. Department of Agriculture estimates Americans added more sugar to their diet every year since the 1970s until 2000. When Americans dropped the added sugar, they turned to sugarlike extracts. The sugar substitute market was estimated to be worth $10.5 billion in 2012, according an analysis by Markets and Markets research firm.

And the market may be growing. Just 18 percent of U.S. adults used low- or no-calorie sweeteners in 2000. Now, 24 percent of adults and 12 percent of children use the sugar substitutes, according to a 2012 review in the American Journal of Clinical Nutrition.

There are even other health benefits attributed to Stevia including a reduction in hyper tension a/k/a high blood pressure. I love Stevia and use it regularly in lieu of sugar. But I do caution that in many respects Stevia is still the new kid on the block and over time there may well be some evidence of negative aspects of Stevia. I am not saying that it will happen that way, but it is often the way something new develops over time. At first it is a blessed miracle, but then researchers start finding a dark side. Again I am not saying that it will happen like that but it could so if you join me and millions of others who have accepted Stevia is our sweetener of choice that is fine, just stay informed.

That's a Wrap

We began by coming to understand that the problem of obesity is far more prevalent today than ever before in our human history. For many, especially amongst woman obesity or being a "a bit over weight" has been more a matter of concern over image rather than fundamental health. So we began by gaining an important understanding that obesity is first and foremost a serious and even potentially deadly health concern.

That awareness I believe helps us move to the next critical step on this road to greater health where it becomes essential that we take ownership of the problem. Trying to ignore the problem and hoping that it will just go away, or making nonsense excuses to ourselves accomplishes absolutely nothing good. Yes, taking ownership of the matter can be difficult and stressful but it is absolutely required for without doing so the problem only keeps getting worse. But what do we do?

That takes us to the two part solution of eating less and moving more. Indeed our food intake, both how much and what kind is about 80% of the story. We need not only to eat a bit less but we must also begin to shift to a far healthier diet if we are regain or perhaps gain for the first time a state of good health. We live in world where the nasty food surrounds us and unfortunately it often does taste great. Dealing with that reality is a tough but absolutely essential task. So I explore with you the concept of good foods versus bad foods and how to measure which foods to choose. Improving our diet can and will make a huge difference in our overall health but frequently going "on a diet" accomplishes nothing good long term.

Next up we get into the area of physical activity. That is an area that has also come under attack in our modern digital world where absolutely everything is controlled by some electronic device leaving us to merely sit and rot in our recliner. Just as making a shift away from bad food to good food takes knowledge and discipline, so does weaning ourselves off of stagnation to positive motion. Yet again it is a critical action in our quest for greater health and longer life.

I also take a long walk through the subject of water for the simple reason that water is well over half of our actual bodies. Since water is so much of our physical being it is very important to really know how to obtain and use the best possible water. It is highly unlikely that even the worst municipal water will cause substantial grave health consequences, but over time exposure to unclean unsafe water can have a deeply damaging impact. So once again it becomes a matter of greater knowledge can lead to better health.

I then had to address what I know would be the thoughts of many and that is my position in all of this is invalid because we all know of people who do indeed live long and seemingly health lives despite their total absence of any concerns over poor eating habits, little exercise and a state or obesity. But to focus on the exceptions while ignoring the widely applicable general rule is a potentially deadly bit of very dangerous self-deception.

Along that path I introduced you to four celebrities. Three of them died at a far too young age primarily due to a very obvious condition of extreme obesity. My only point being not a personal slam against these three very talented young men, but rather the revelation that no amount of fame or fortune will protect you from the powerful realities of life. The fourth celebrity I chose was to illustrate that it is indeed possible to turn around an unhealthy lifestyle and gain or perhaps regain a far more healthy and happy life.

And now just for further benefit immediately following this wrap I have added some very important web links for your further exploration. In a very fundamental way I really do believe that what is presented here is to a very large extent all you need to turn your life around. That said it is also true that greater knowledge gives you more and stronger tools for making the changes you need to make. So by all means check out what follows and then may you enjoy a magnificent, long and healthy life free of all disease and filled with positive energy.

Ron Irwin

Other Resources

Even though I did boldly claim that this is the only book you will ever need to deal with reshaping your lifestyle, losing weight and living better and longer, the truth of the matter is that there are several other resources you may well find useful. Here are a few links to other writings and websites you may well find useful.

I already mentioned Neal Barnard MD's very helpful book *Dr. Neal Barnard's Program for Reversing Type II Diabetes* but it deserves further mention. Dr. Barnard's approach is essentially a vegan approach to diet and frankly I did not and will not totally follow his track. That said he does offer so much solid science based information, real world solutions to many serious health problems that it is a great idea to spend a little time taking a closer look at the thoughts, teachings and ideas of Neal Barnard, MD. Here is a great place to start.

http://www.pcrm.org/media/experts/neal-barnard-diabetes-book

From the Food Network comes a resource well worth your time. It is several Vegan recipes and while I will say again that I cannot quite take myself fully into the Vegan camp the fact of the matter is that Vegan recipes do offer several great healthy eating options. So you may want to spend a little time checking out this website.

http://www.foodnetwork.com/topics/vegan.html

And here are nine more Vegan recipes from Good Housekeeping. By looking at all of these recipe ideas you will begin to develop your own sense of how to prepare meals that are not only devoid of most of the "Unwanteds" but also tasty and satisfying.

http://www.goodhousekeeping.com/food-recipes/g807/vegan-recipes/

Less "hardcore" than the Vegan approach is the Vegetarian approach. The Vegetarian diet has most of the same health aspects of more severe Vegan diet but they do provide a wider range of options. So here then is another resource worthy of your time. This is from Cooking Light. Just the title is inviting.

http://www.cookinglight.com/food/top-rated-recipes/best-vegetarian-recipes

Here is another great source of recipe ideas from Eating Well. Again you should not only follow some of the more appealing recipes but also use them as a base line as you begin to experiment with your ideas.

http://www.eatingwell.com/recipes_menus/vegetarian_recipes

If you have been a couch potato for a long time it is possible that even though you would like to exercise more you have long forgotten the best ways to get in gear. So why not start with this offering from Web MD.

http://www.webmd.com/fitness-exercise/

I really love this article from FamilyDoctor.org because it focuses on the need to make regular exercise a habit. Once that is accomplished everything just keeps getting better. Take a look.

http://familydoctor.org/familydoctor/en/prevention-wellness/exercise-fitness/exercise-basics/the-exercise-habit.html

This offering from Mayo Clinic is also something you need to read and heed because it focuses on the main and very important real health benefits of regular exercise. Odds are you will never compete in the Olympics but you absolutely can successfully attack several diseases, achieve a better mood and get more energy. Here is what the Mayo Clinic has to say on the subject.

http://www.mayoclinic.org/healthy-lifestyle/fitness/in-depth/exercise/art-20048389

And if I still haven't motivated you to get your butt in gear here is an article from Woman's Day on ten exercises for better sex.

http://www.womansday.com/relationships/sex-tips/advice/a2072/10-exercises-for-better-sex-112752/

At the risk of seeming like a "downer" I cannot avoid a little more discussion about Diabetes because it so darn miserable and very much preventable but it is heavily linked with obesity. So here is another article from Obisty.org that further explores the subject. The best time to get the fact about diabetes is BEFORE you get it.

http://www.obesity.org/resources-for/your-weight-and-diabetes.htm

And while I know you don't really want to read this stuff because it can be both unpleasant and scary, it is extremely important that you become fully aware. So here is one more article/website dealing with the subject of diabetes and obesity. This is from MedicinNet.com.

http://www.medicinenet.com/script/main/art.asp?articlekey=39840

Okay now I have to offer you one more very scary bit of detailed information, this time on Congestive Heart Failure because yet again while obesity does not necessarily CAUSE Congestive Heart Failure the two conditions tend to go hand in hand. And Congestive Heart Failure is often deadly so do invest just wee bit of time getting the fundamental information from WebMD.

http://www.webmd.com/heart-disease/guide-heart-failure